Bone Broth

[MATTHEW LIVINGSTON]

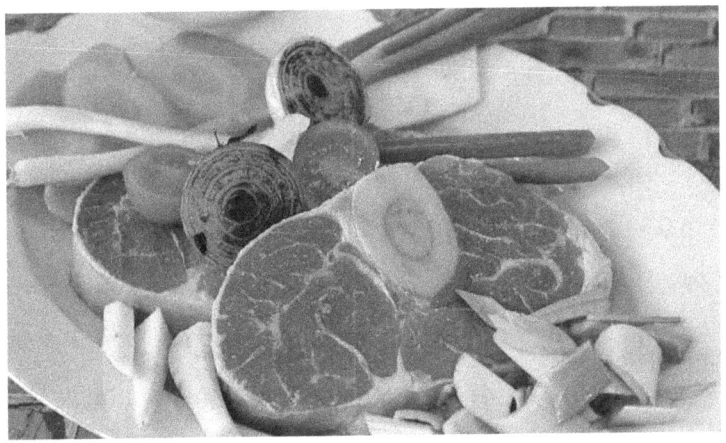

Legal & Disclaimer

The information contained in this book and its contents is not designed to replace or take the place of any form of medical or professional advice; and is not meant to replace the need for independent medical, financial, legal or other professional advice or services, as may be required. The content and information in this book have been provided for educational and entertainment purposes only.

The content and information contained in this book have been compiled from sources deemed reliable, and it is accurate to the best of the Author's knowledge, information, and belief. However, the Author cannot guarantee its accuracy and validity and cannot be held liable for any errors and/or omissions. Further, changes are periodically made to this book as and when needed. Where appropriate and/or necessary, you must consult a professional (including but not limited to your doctor, attorney, financial advisor or such other professional advisor) before using any of the suggested remedies, techniques, or information in this book.

Upon using the contents and information contained in this book, you agree to hold harmless the Author from and against any damages, costs, and expenses, including any legal fees potentially resulting from the application of any of the information provided by this book. This disclaimer applies to any loss, damages or injury caused by the use and application, whether directly or indirectly, of any advice or information presented, whether for breach of contract, tort, negligence, personal injury, criminal intent, or under any other cause of action.

You agree to accept all risks of using the information presented inside this book.

You agree that by continuing to read this book, where appropriate and/or necessary, you shall consult a professional (including but not limited to your doctor, attorney, or financial advisor or such other advisor as needed) before using any of the suggested remedies, techniques, or information in this book.

Table of Contents

Introduction

Bone broth is delicious and healthy at the same time, so it makes sense why you should be interested in incorporating it more often in the diet. It might surprise you to find out but there are numerous uses for bone broth in the diet, going beyond the idea of soup and stew (which you are probably accustomed to). So, let's see how you can consume more bone broth, enjoying the innovative suggestions gathered especially for you.

Bone broth as a morning beverage

For many people, coffee is the ideal morning beverage. However, if you are looking to make a change, you can try out a cup of hot bone broth as your morning beverage. You can add some spices and herbs, enjoying your new choice to the fullest.

Bone broth as soup/stew base

This is indeed one of the most common uses of bone broth, helping you make a delicious soup or stew. All you have to do is head the bone broth, adding meat and veggies, thus obtaining a delicious meal. The bone broth can successfully replace the traditional bouillon cube, so make sure you give it a try. You can even take this meal, in a thermos, at work or on the road.

Bone broth for pasta and rice

You can easily add flavor to many pasta or rice dishes by cooking them in bone broth, instead of water.

Bone broth for baby food

When you prepare vegetable puree for your baby, you can easily replace the necessary quantity of water with bone broth. In this way, you will add flavor to the pureed veggies, providing your baby with a new and delicious taste.

Bone broth for mashed potatoes or cauliflower

If you want to add flavor to your mashed potatoes/cauliflower, all you have to do is use bone broth instead of milk. Apart from adding flavor, the bone broth will also moisten the mashed potatoes or cauliflower, with a guaranteed creamy texture.

Bone broth, an essential ingredient for delicious sauces

Some of the most delicious sauces can be prepared by substituting water with bone broth. You can even use it, in order to prepare gravy; you can begin by reducing the bone broth, seasoning it with salt and pepper. Then, add a little bit of tapioca starch and mix well, enjoying your newly-made gravy (which is grain free, another benefit to enjoy). Many people resort to bone broth for the making of white sauces as well, sometimes substituting milk (valid for cheese-based sauces). And, remember, bone broth is an excellent ingredient to add to a salad dressing or dipping sauce (unique flavor and taste).

Bone broth, frozen

An ingenious idea refers to pouring bone broth in the ice cube tray and placing it in the freezer. You can then use the bone broth cubes, in order to prepare delicious breakfast smoothies. This is especially valid for hot summer days when you do not feel like eating anything else for breakfast. Plus, the bone broth cube will deliver a healthy portion of proteins, necessary for a good start in the day.

Bone broth and sautéed/steamed veggies

We all love to eat sautéed or steamed veggies, as these are healthy and chock full of vitamins. Well, if you want to make them even more delicious, all you have to do is add one cube of frozen bone broth. For example, you can use bone broth when you are making steamed broccoli, enjoying the new combination of flavors.

Bone broth and refried beans

In the situation that you are thinking about refrying beans, you might want to use bone broth instead of water. Indeed, water is commonly used to thin out the beans but using bone broth will add even more flavor, so be sure to consider it.

Bone broth for egg-based dishes

Scrambled eggs represent the ideal breakfast choice, with milk being often used to make them fluffier. However, if you want to add a little bit of flavor to your eggs, consider using bone broth instead of milk. The same goes for other egg-based dishes, such as frittatas, omelets or quiches, where the required liquids can be replaced with bone broth.

Bone broth and tomato sauce

If you are going to prepare a dish that requires tomato sauce, such as chili, you can use bone broth to dilute it. In this way, the dish is going to be lighter and not as heavy on the stomach. Moreover, the bone broth will add a unique flavor to your tomato sauce, complementing the rest of the ingredients used for the making of the respective dish.

These are only a couple of ways in which you can incorporate bone broth in the diet. As you have probably figured out, bone broth can be used to dilute certain ingredients but also add a unique flavor to your dishes. In the following chapter, you will discover a number of exciting recipes that are prepared with bone broth as an essential ingredient.

Chapter 1: Health Benefits of the Bone Broth Diet

The bone broth diet is a revolutionary method of losing weight, combining mini-fasting with regular eating (from a list of allowed foods). Scientists have been talking about the health benefits of fasting for many years now but it was only recently that people have discovered them. Let's look at a few important health benefits of the bone broth diet.

1. Promotes healthy joints

Why is this important? When individuals age, their joints experience wear and tear as cartilage diminishes. Bone broth provides the collagen from the animal parts that can be readily absorbable to help restore lost cartilage.

Bond broth also provides an extremely important substance known as gelatin. In our bodies, gelatin acts as a cushion between bones which allows bones to glide without friction between joints. Gelatin is also involved in maintaining healthy bone density.

2. Promotes a healthy gut

The gelatin found in bone broth is extremely beneficial for our gut. Gelatin has been demonstrated to aid in strengthening gut lining, decreasing sensitivities to certain allergens and types of foods, aiding in the increasing probiotics, and supporting healthy inflammation levels in the digestive tract.

Studies have also shown that supplementing with collagen can be extremely beneficial for one's digestive tract as the amino acids in collagen help form tissues in colon and gastrointestinal tract.

3. Promotes beautiful skin

The collagen in bone broth promotes the production of substances within the body that are needed for maintaining a youthful appearance like elastin. The supplementation of collagen has been known to decrease cellulite, wrinkles, and puffiness. Studies have also shown that collagen promotes skin firmness, elasticity, and moisture.

4. Supports Immune System Function

The positive effect bone broth has on the gut helps support a healthy immune system functioning by preventing leaky gut. Leaky gut is a dysfunctional condition where food particles pass through openings in the intestine and enter the bloodstream. As a result, the immune system detects these particles and becomes hyperactive causing various bodily dysfunctions.

5. Aids in Detoxification

In modern society, individuals come into contact with a wide array of toxins. Bone broth is a very effective detoxifying agent as it contains both potassium and glycine, both of which support cellular and liver detoxification. Bone broth also has sulphur and glutathione which act as antioxidants in the body.

Paleo, Juicing, and Detoxing

The bone broth diet is a very important part of a paleo regiment. Paleo eaters, as you may know, are supposed to fast / detox two days a week. Traditionally, this is done through either juicing with vegetable juice or abstaining from food altogether. The purpose of this is to reset the body's metabolism, decrease inflammation, reduce blood glucose levels, and help you lose weight by burning ketones for energy versus glucose.

The problem with fasting /detoxing/juicing is that anybody who does it knows that you suffer from energy loss-related issues. For at least a few days starting out, people on the paleo, ketogenic and similar diets are sometimes barely able to function at work. As for people who do long-term liquid diets for rapid weight loss—it's a great strategy for losing weight but it can leave you feeling really crappy for a long time.

Bone brothing (that's my new verb form) to some extent solves this problem. Most bone broth recipes are high in protein, which solves the problem that juicers/detoxers face where their energy levels crash. It's possible to detox or juice using a mixture of bone broth and traditional juicing recipes, and feel MUCH better throughout your diet.

For this reason, I now believe bone broth is a cornerstone to not only a successful paleo protocol, but also a successful weight loss strategy. A girlfriend of mine went from 300 lbs to 135 lbs in 4 months switching entirely to a liquid diet. This is hard to do and requires a lot of effort and discipline on anyone's part; however, the addition of bone broth helped her survive because the protein kept her diet balanced.

This is also important for anyone who wants to fast / juice who suffers from blood sugar related issues. If this is you, consult with your doctor about implementing a weight loss plan that substitutes fruit and veggie juice with bone broth.

How to Get Started

It's time to make our poor vegan friends cringe by making friends with the local supermarket butcher. Since we're a spoiled Western country, we tend to neglect parts of animals that aren't palatable by Western standards—the feet, throats or other edible but discarded areas. These, however, often make the best collagen-rich areas of the animal to make broth from. You can likely buy bulk supplies of this stuff for a relatively low price at any supermarket butcher. Or go to an Asian grocer. People in countries like Thailand make soups out of these parts all day long.

It's recommended for most broths to be frozen if you're not going to immediately consume them. It's not suggested to keep any mason jars of broth in the regular fridge for more than a week. Frozen jars, however, can be kept for a long time (a year or longer). However, it would be silly to wait for months to have your broth. If I freeze broth it will be used a few weeks after I finish the other batch. The point is just to stock up a bulk supply by consolidating your cooking time.

Next, when consuming bone broth, a few pointers to keep in mind:

- Have bone broth with water, when possible.

- Mix up days that you are fasting/consuming only bone broth. Don't go to a strict liquid diet without consulting a doctor as this can be pretty intense. Further, don't limit your intake to only bone broth—you need a healthy mix of juicing, as well.

- During fasting periods, you can substitute breakfast and lunch with bone broth but have a light meal for dinner (something with green vegetables)

- Limit desserts in general. Especially avoid during fasting days.

Chapter 2: Recipes

Appetizers

Buffalo Wings

Preparation Time: 10 minutes

Cooking Time: 2 hours

Serves: 6

Ingredients

- Chili pepper sauce, 1 bottle, 300 ml
- 2 teaspoons dried oregano
- 2 tablespoons butter
- 2 teaspoons garlic powder
- 2 teaspoons onion powder
- 1 tablespoon Worcestershire sauce
- 500 grams of chicken wings

Preparation

- Preheat the oven to 180 degrees C

- Place the butter chili sauce, Worcestershire sauce, garlic powder, onion powder, and oregano. Allow simmering for five minutes.
- Place your chicken wings into a glass baking dish and pour the sauce mix over it. For 2 hours cover with foil.
- Reduce the heat to 100 degrees C and uncover. Cook for 2 more hours. Take out of the oven and serve.

Nutritional info

Calories: 78

Total fat: 1.7

Saturated fat: 0.5

Cholesterol: 38 mg

Sodium: 138 mg

Potassium: 185 mg

Total Carbohydrates: 0.8 g

Protein: 14.0 g

Teriyaki Chicken Wings

Preparation Time: 2 hours, 10 minutes

Cooking Time: 4 hours

Serves: 10

Ingredients

- 2 kilos chicken wings
- 2 tablespoons brown sugar
- 1 teaspoon garlic powder
- 1 teaspoon ground ginger
- 1 cup of water
- 1 cup of soy sauce
- ½ cup pineapple juice
- 2 tablespoons vegetable oil

Preparation

- Except for the chicken, mix the other ingredients. Once they are all mixed, add the chicken and toss it gently until it is well coated with the mixture. Put it away in the refrigerator to marinate for about 2 hours

- Remove from the marinade and place in a baking dish. Baste with some of the marinades.
- At 180 degrees C, bake for two hours. Uncover, and finish off for fifteen minutes.

Nutritional info

Calories: 68

Total fat: 1.9

Saturated fat: 0

Cholesterol: 24 mg

Sodium: 1050 mg

Potassium: 216 mg

Total Carbohydrates: 3.8 g

Protein: 9.2 g

Pigs in a Blanket

Preparation Time: 10 minutes

Cooking Time: 1 hour 30 minutes

Serves: 10

Ingredients

- 300 grams streaky bacon
- 300 grams beef cocktail sausages
- ½ cup brown sugar

Preparation

- Preheat oven to 160 degrees C
- Wrap each cocktail sausage with a rasher of bacon. Hold in place using a toothpick. Arrange on a prepared baking sheet.
- Generously sprinkle sugar over the wrapped sausages
- Bake for forty minutes in the preheated oven or until the sugar is bubbly.
- Reduce the heat to 100 degrees C and continue cooking for one hour.

Nutritional info

Calories: 114

Total fat: 2.5

Saturated fat: 0.9

Cholesterol: 52 mg

Sodium: 58 mg

Potassium: 366 mg

Total Carbohydrates: 3.1 g

Protein: 18.9 g

Bacon, Beef and Cheese Dip

Preparation Time: 15 minutes

Cooking Time: 1 hours 10 minutes

Serves: 8

Ingredients

- Olive oil
- 250 grams minced beef
- Six rashers of bacon
- 1 cup cheddar cheese, grated
- 1 cup cream cheese
- 2 teaspoons fresh parsley, finely chopped
- 1 can tomatoes, chopped
- 1 red capsicum, chopped finely

Preparation

- Grill the bacon on a frying pan until it is crisp. Remove from the heat and drain on paper towels. When drained, crumble into fine pieces.

- Place oil in a pan on medium heat. Add in the ground beef and brown well. Drain any excess oil.
- Add in the cheddar cheese and cream cheese and mix well. Add the bacon, then the tomatoes.
- Place in a slow cooker on low heat, and leave to cook gently for one hour. Stir occasionally as it gets hot and bubbly.
- Stir in the parsley and sprinkle the reserved bacon for garnish. Serve as a dip with nachos and veggie strips.

Nutritional info

Calories: 116

Total fat: 2.4

Saturated fat: 0.8

Cholesterol: 47 mg

Sodium: 69 mg

Potassium: 421 mg

Total Carbohydrates: 5.3 g

Protein: 17.7 g

Ketchup Meatballs with a Touch of Beer

Preparation Time: 15 minutes

Cooking Time: 2 hours, 30 minutes

Serves: 8

Ingredients

- 750 grams ground beef
- One can beer
- 200 ml ketchup
- 1 teaspoon sliced garlic
- 1 large onion, finely chopped
- Salt and Pepper to season

Preparation

- Preheat your oven to 150 degrees Celsius
- Place the ketchup and beer in a medium saucepan and allow to simmer over medium heat. Reduce to half the quantity.

- Combine the onions, garlic and minced beef. Season with salt and pepper.
- Shape the mincemeat into meatballs, and place in a baking dish.
- Pour the ketchup and beer reduction over the meatballs.
- For 2 hours, bake. Serve in a rich, sticky, thickened sauce.

Nutritional info:

Calories: 152

Total fat: 4.8

Saturated fat: 1.7

Cholesterol: 66 mg

Sodium: 335 mg

Potassium: 380 mg

Total Carbohydrates: 4.4 g

Protein: 22.0 g

Crab and Artichoke Spread on Toast

Preparation Time: 10 minutes

Cooking Time: 1 hour

Serves: 4

Ingredients

- One cup crab meat, flaky
- One can artichoke hearts, chopped
- Juice of one lemon
- Three tablespoons parmesan cheese, grated
- Four spring onions, sliced
- One red capsicum, cut into
- Four medium green onions. Slice them up to about 1/4 cup
- A red bell pepper. Cut into wide wedges
- 8 slices of wholemeal bread
- 250 grams of cream cheese

Preparation

- Take a large slow cooker and place all the ingredients within it, except for the bell peppers and wholemeal bread.
- For one hour, bake and stir
- Serve in the capsicum wedges and over the sliced bread.

Nutritional info:

Calories: 122

Total fat: 3.0

Saturated fat: 0.9

Cholesterol: 60 mg

Sodium: 57 mg

Potassium: 303 mg

Total Carbohydrates: 0.8 g

Protein: 21.9 g

Sticky Cocktail Sausages

Preparation Time: 10 minutes

Cooking Time: 2 hours

Serves: 10

Ingredients

- 500 grams smoked sausage, thickly sliced
- 2 tablespoons packed brown sugar
- 1 small finely chopped onion
- Small bottle of chili sauce
- 1/2 cup bourbon

Preparation

- Place a large skillet over medium heat.
- Add your cut sausages and let them cook for about 2 minutes on each side or until they are browned. Remove and drain on towels.
- Prepare a medium slow cooker by spraying cooking spray. Mix the chili sauce, bourbon,

onion and sugar together in a small bowl. Add to the slow cooker and heat through. Add the sausages and coat with the sauce.

- For two hours, cook. The sauce should turn thick and sticky.
- Add a dash of beef broth is the sauce is too thick to prevent sticking.

Nutritional info

Calories: 155

Total fat: 5.9

Saturated fat: 2.1

Cholesterol: 72 mg

Sodium: 476 mg

Potassium: 314 mg

Total Carbohydrates: 1.2 g

Protein: 22.7 g

Sweet and Sour Meatballs

Preparation Time: 15 minutes

Cooking Time: 3 hours 30 minutes

Serves: 8

Ingredients

- One kilo minced beef

- One onion, finely chopped

- One Egg

- Salt and pepper to taste

- 300 ml of chili sauce

- ½ cup grape jelly

Preparation

- To create the meatballs, combine the beef, onion, egg, and seasoning in a large bowl until well combined. Shape into small meatballs.
- In a slow cooker, place the chili sauce, grape jelly, and juice from one lemon. Add the meatballs and combine gentle.
- Leave on low heat to cook gently for 3 hours, then serve.

Nutritional info*:*

Calories: 95

Total fat: 1.7

Saturated fat: 0.5

Cholesterol: 32 mg

Sodium: 300 mg

Potassium: 283 mg

Total Carbohydrates: 7.2 g

Protein: 12.8 g

Bean and Cheese Dip

Preparation Time: 5 minutes

Cooking Time: 1 hours

Serves: 4

Ingredients

- One can of refried beans
- One small can jalapeno peppers
- One pack of mild Mexican cheese, cut into cubes
- One kilo Tortilla Chips to serve
- Slow cooker liners

Preparation

- Place the slow cooker liners inside a slow cooker, making sure that all the sides are well covered.
- Place the beans, chilies, and cheese into the cooker. Gently combine until mixed through.

- For one hour, cook as you stir occasionally to ensure the cheese remains smooth.

- Serve with tortilla chips for a cheesy treat.

Nutritional info

Calories: 204

Total fat: 4.1

Saturated fat: 1.4

Cholesterol: 83 mg

Sodium: 86 mg

Potassium: 622 mg

Total Carbohydrates: 10.6 g

Protein: 30.2 g

Sauerkraut Dip

Preparation Time: 10 minutes

Cooking Time: 50 minutes

Serves: 4

Ingredients

- One 400g jar of Sauerkraut
- 200 grams of cream cheese
- 1 cup Swiss cheese, grated
- 1 cup corned beef, shredded
- 1/3 cup thousand Island dressing

Preparation

- Combine the sauerkraut, cheese, beef, and dressing. For about 45 minutes, cook. Make sure to stir occasionally as the cheese melts.
- Serve with some crackers or crusty bread.

Nutritional info

Calories: 106

Total fat: 2.6

Saturated fat: 0.7

Cholesterol: 43 mg

Sodium: 74 mg

Potassium: 243 mg

Total Carbohydrates: 4.0 g

Protein: 16.1 g

Chapter 3: Main Dishes

Roast with Cranberries

Preparation Time: 10 minutes

Cooking Time: 8 hours, 15 minutes

Serves: 6

Ingredients

- 1.5 kg beef chuck roast
- One packet onion soup mix
- 2 cups beef stock
- 2 large spoons plain flour
- 2 large spoons butter
- One can cranberry sauce, jellied

Preparation

- Put the roast on top, and top with beef stock and cranberry sauce.
- Cover and cook for 8 hours on a low heat setting.

- Once the roast is cooked, drain the juices and keep separate.
- In a small pan, whisk together butter and flour, and slowly add the reserved juices to create a thick gravy. Serve with the roast.

Nutritional info

Calories: 117

Total fat: 5.2

Saturated fat: 3.1

Cholesterol: 45 mg

Sodium: 725 mg

Potassium: 231 mg

Total Carbohydrates: 1.0 g

Protein: 16.1 g

Buffalo Chicken Sandwiches

Preparation Time: 10 minutes

Cooking Time: 2 hours 30 minutes

Serves: 4

Ingredients

- 4 skinless, boneless chicken breast, halved
- 2 tablespoons butter
- 1 cup chicken stock
- 4 bread rolls, cut lengthwise
- ½ cup ketchup
- ¼ cup barbecue sauce
- ½ cup ranch dressing

Preparation

- Melt the butter in a slow cooker, and lightly brown the chicken breasts. Add the chicken stock and leave to cook for 1 hour.

- After an hour, add the ketchup and barbecue sauce. Allow to cook on low heat for
- another hour.
- Use the chicken to fill in the bread rolls. Use any remaining sauce as a dip.

Nutritional info

Calories: 123

Total fat: 3.0

Saturated fat: 1.0

Cholesterol: 35 mg

Sodium: 38 mg

Potassium: 225 mg

Total Carbohydrates: 10.3 g

Protein: 13.4 g

The Ultimate Pot Roast

Preparation Time: 10 minutes

Cooking Time: 4 hours 20 minutes

Serves: 8

Ingredients

- 2.5 kilos of chuck steak beef
- 2 cups beef bone broth
- Two cans of mushroom soup
- A pack of onion soup

Preparation

- In a slow cooker, combine the mushroom soup, onion soup and beef bone broth. Place your pot roast into a slow cooker and coat cover it well with the soup mixture

- Cook on low heat for 4 hours. If liquid reduces and the meat cannot be separated with a fork, add some more soup and cook for another hour.
- Serve on a bed of buttery tagliatelle.

Nutritional info:

Calories: 77

Total fat: 1.9

Saturated fat: 0.6

Cholesterol: 28 mg

Sodium: 33 mg

Potassium: 193 mg

Total Carbohydrates: 4.7 g

Protein: 10.5 g

Peppery Chinese Steaks

Preparation Time: 20 minutes

Cooking Time: 2 hours 10 minutes

Serves: 4

Ingredients

- ¼ cup olive oil
- One kilo beef sirloin, cut into 2-inch strips
- One cup beef bone broth
- One can tomatoes, chopped
- Two large green bell peppers, chopped roughly
- One teaspoon garlic powder
- One teaspoon sugar
- ¼ cup of soy sauce
- Salt and Pepper

Preparation

- Elevate the flavor by sprinkling strips.

- Place the beef into a slow cooker, and add the broth and tomatoes after heating oil.
- Add in all the vegetables, soy sauce, sugar, and seasoning.
- Stir, and cover the cooked. Keep on low heat for two hours and serve with steamed rice.

Nutritional info

Calories: 149

Total fat: 4.2

Saturated fat: 1.6

Cholesterol: 54 mg

Sodium: 1732 mg

Potassium: 406 mg

Total Carbohydrates: 7.1 g

Protcin: 20.0 g

Patience Baby Back Ribs

Preparation Time: 10 minutes

Cooking Time: 4 hours 20 minutes

Serves: 8

Ingredients

- 2 kilos baby back ribs
- 300 ml barbecue sauce
- One clove of garlic, sliced
- One onion, finely sliced
- Salt and pepper to season
- 1 cup beef bone broth

Preparation

- Rub the ribs with salt and pepper to season them.
- Take a slow cooker and pour in the stock. Layer the ribs in the slow cooker and top them up with garlic and onion.

- Cook on medium heat for 4 hours
- Preheat your oven to 190 degrees C
- Transfer the ribs to a prepared baking sheet, leaving out the garlic and onions. Coat them with the barbeque sauce and bake in the preheated oven until the sauce caramelizes and sticks to the ribs. This should be about 20 minutes.

Nutritional info

Calories: 68

Total fat: 1.5

Saturated fat: 0.5

Cholesterol: 20 mg

Sodium: 1577 mg

Potassium: 182 mg

Total Carbohydrates: 6.2 g

Protein: 7.6 g

Melt in your Mouth Pork Tenderloin

Preparation Time: 10 minutes

Cooking Time: 3 hours

Serves: 8

Ingredients

- One kilo pork tenderloin
- One pack dry onion soup
- One cup chicken bone broth
- 1/3 cup soy sauce
- ½ cup red wine
- 2 cloves garlic, sliced

Preparation

- Add in the bone broth, red wine and soy sauce over the top. Make sure that the liquid covers the pork.
- Add the garlic to the slow cooker. Cover and keep cooking on low for 3 hours.

Nutritional info

Calories: 130

Total fat: 5.1

Saturated fat: 1.8

Cholesterol: 51 mg

Sodium: 437 mg

Potassium: 287 mg

Total Carbohydrates: 3.4 g

Protein: 17.5 g

Pepperoncini Beef

Preparation Time: 10 minutes

Cooking Time: 8 hours

Serves: 8

Ingredients

- One and a half kilos beef chuck roast
- 4 cups beef bone broth
- 8 bread rolls, sliced lengthwise
- 4 tablespoons pepperoncini
- 4 cloves of garlic, sliced
- 8 slices provolone cheese
- Salt and Pepper to season

Preparation

- Take your roast and make small incisions all around it. Place slices of garlic into each of the incisions.

52

- Then, place the roast in a slow cooker and add the beef bone broth. Season. Cover and cook on for 8 hours.
- Separate the beef with a fork to get shreds. Fill the bread rolls with the beef and top with pepperoncini.
- Top with the cheese slices and serve.

Nutritional info

Calories: 121

Total fat: 4.7

Saturated fat: 1.4

Cholesterol: 41 mg

Sodium: 52 mg

Potassium: 322 mg

Total Carbohydrates: 4.7 g

Protein: 14.g

Pulled Beef

Preparation Time: 15 minutes

Cooking Time: 8 hours

Serves: 6

Ingredients

- One kilo rump roast
- 4 cups beef stock
- Basil, oregano, parsley, onion powder, and garlic salt.
- Salt and pepper to taste
- One bay leaf
- Italian Salad Dressing

Preparation

- Seasoning, dry herbs and bay leaf. Add two tablespoons of Italian salad dressing mix. Combine well and bring them to a boil.

- Add the beef and ensure that it is fully covered by the sauce. Set on low heat and cook for eight hours. Finally shred the meat.

Nutritional info:

Calories: 67

Total fat: 2.0

Saturated fat: 0.8

Cholesterol: 28 mg

Sodium: 293 mg

Potassium: 173 mg

Total Carbohydrates: 2.1 g

Protein: 9.8 g

Slowly Cooked Honey Garlic Chicken

Preparation Time: 10 minutes

Cooking Time: 4 hours

Serves: 5

Ingredients

- Olive oil
- 5 chicken breasts, boneless and skinless
- 200 grams pineapple tidbits
- 2 garlic cloves, crushed
- 1-inch ginger, minced
- 3/4 cup chicken bone broth
- 3/4 cup honey
- 3/4 cup soy sauce
- ¼ cup ketchup

Preparation

- Heat oil and cook the chicken breasts just until evenly browned on all sides.
- Transfer the chicken into a slow cooker.
- Combine the soy sauce, honey, ketchup, ginger, garlic, and the chicken bone broth. Pour the mixture into the slow cooker.
- Cover the cooker and cook 4 hours on low heat.
- Stir in pineapple tidbits just before serving.

Nutritional info:

Calories: 99

Total fat: 2.6

Saturated fat: 1.0

Cholesterol: 36 mg

Sodium: 46 mg

Potassium: 275 mg

Total Carbohydrates: 5.5 g

Protein: 12.9 g

Barbeque Shredded Beef

Preparation Time: 10 minutes

Cooking Time: 2 hours

Serves: 4

Ingredients

- 1 kg chuck steak, boneless
- 1 onion, finely chopped
- 1 can tomatoes, chopped
- 1/3 cup vinegar
- 1/3 cup brown sugar
- ¼ teaspoon soy sauce
- Salt and pepper

Preparation

- Place all ingredients in the barbecue, covered with foil, and cook for 2 hours.

- Uncover, and continue cooking for one hour. Then it is ready to serve.

Nutritional info

Calories: 179

Total fat: 5.4

Saturated fat: 1.9

Cholesterol: 71 mg

Sodium: 1072 mg

Potassium: 385 mg

Total Carbohydrates: 6.5 g

Protein: 25.5 g

Rubbed Beef

Preparation Time: 20 minutes

Cooking Time: 4 hours

Serves: 6

Ingredients

- 500 grams' chuck steak, boneless
- 2 teaspoons onion and garlic powder
- Salt and pepper

Preparation

- Rub the beef with the powder, salt, and pepper, making sure it is well rubbed in.
- Place in a barbeque, on a piece of foil.
- Cover and allow to cook for 4 hours.
- Rest the meat for 20 minutes before serving.

Nutritional info

Calories: 77

Total fat: 2.5

Saturated fat: 0.8

Cholesterol: 28 mg

Sodium: 350 mg

Potassium: 197 mg

Total Carbohydrates: 4.3 g

Protein: 9.5 g

Ground Beef Barbecue

Preparation Time: 10 minutes

Cooking Time: 5 hours

Serves: 4

Ingredients

- 500 grams minced beef
- 2 garlic cloves, sliced
- 1 large onion, chopped
- 1 tablespoon mustard
- 1 cup beef bone broth
- 1 tablespoon apple cider vinegar
- Dash of ketchup
- Salt and pepper

Preparation

- Place all the ingredients in a baking dish and mix well.

- Place this dish in the barbecue, and cook for 5 hours on low heat. Once every hour stir to prevent sticking.
- Make sure to keep covered so that it does not dry out.

Nutritional info

Calories: 125

Total fat: 3.7

Saturated fat: 1.3

Cholesterol: 41 mg

Sodium: 64 mg

Potassium: 356 mg

Total Carbohydrates: 9.1 g

Protein: 13.8 g

Pork Barbeque

Preparation Time: 10 minutes

Cooking Time: 1 hour

Serves: 4

Ingredients

- 4 pork chops
- Lemon Juice
- Dash of Honey
- Salt and Pepper to season

Preparation

- Combine all the ingredients together
- Place on the barbeque on low heat, and leave to cook for one hour.
- Turn the pork chops over at the half-hour mark.

Nutritional info:

Calories: 76

Total fat: 2.9

Saturated fat: 1.0

Cholesterol: 36 mg

Sodium: 372 mg

Potassium: 158 mg

Total Carbohydrates: 0.6 g

Protein: 11.4 g

BBQ Pork for Sandwiches

Preparation Time: 3 hours

Cooking Time: 6 hours 30 minutes

Serves: 6

Ingredients

- 500 ml of chicken bone broth
- 2 kilos pork ribs
- 100 ml barbecue sauce
- 100 ml honey
- Salt and pepper to taste

Preparation

- Combine all ingredients in a bowl and marinade in the fridge for 3 hours.
- Place in a baking dish on the barbecue, covered, and cook on low heat for 6 hours.
- Remove and return the meat to the barbecue in the dish, uncovered, for 30 minutes.
- Serve as a sandwich filling.

Nutritional info

Calories: 164

Total fat: 7.6

Saturated fat: 1.7

Cholesterol: 34 mg

Sodium: 310 mg

Potassium: 303 mg

Total Carbohydrates: 12.0 g

Protein: 12.8 g

Honey Ribs

Preparation Time: 3 hours

Cooking Time: 6 hours 30 minutes

Serves: 6

Ingredients

- 300 ml beef bone broth
- ¼ cup honey
- 1 tablespoon mustard
- 2 tablespoon barbeque sauce
- ¼ cup of soy sauce
- 1.5 kilos baby back pork ribs

Preparation

- Place all the ingredients in a baking dish and marinade for 4 hours in the fridge.
- Leave outside to rest and reach room temperature for 30 minutes.

- Place in the barbeque on low heat and cook for six hours.
- Slice the risk, leaving meat on the bone, and serve.

Nutritional info

Calories: 38

Total fat: 3.1

Saturated fat: 1.1

Cholesterol: 36 mg

Sodium: 46 mg

Potassium: 213 mg

Total Carbohydrates: 13.9 g

Protein: 12.7 g

Barbecued Beef

Preparation Time: 4 hours

Cooking Time: 6 hours

Serves: 4

Ingredients

- 1 kilo chuck steak, boneless
- 250 ml ketchup
- ¼ cup Worcestershire sauce
- 2 tablespoons brown sugar
- 2 tablespoons vinegar
- 1 tablespoon mustard
- Dash of garlic powder
- Salt and pepper

Preparations

- Mix all ingredients well. Marinade for four hours in the fridge.

- Put the steak on the barbecue on low heat and reserve marinade. Cover and roast for 5 hours.
- Add the reserved marinade to the steak and cook for another 15 minutes.
- Place in a bowl and pull apart using a fork.

Nutritional info:

Calories: 62

Total fat: 2.0

Saturated fat: 0.7

Cholesterol: 22 mg

Sodium: 327 mg

Potassium: 197 mg

Total Carbohydrates: 3.7 g

Protein: 7.5 g

Little Smokies

Preparation Time: 5 minutes

Cooking Time: 1 hours

Serves: 4

Ingredients

- 500 grams smokies sausages
- 2 tablespoon ketchup
- 1 tablespoon barbecue sauce
- 1 tablespoon brown sugar
- 1 tablespoon Worcestershire sauce

Preparation

- Coat the smokies sausages with all the other ingredients.
- Place in the barbecue and cook on low heat for one hour.
- Serve on their own or with potatoes.

Nutritional info

Calories: 156

Total fat: 4.7

Saturated fat: 1.7

Cholesterol: 55 mg

Sodium: 2425 mg

Potassium: 355 mg

Total Carbohydrates: 8.7 g

Protein: 19.3 g

Pulled Chicken Barbecue

Preparation Time: 5 minutes

Cooking Time: 3 hours

Serves: 6

Ingredients

- 6 chicken breasts, boneless and skinless
- 300 ml barbecue sauce
- 600 ml chicken bone broth
- 100 ml Italian vinaigrette
- 2 tablespoons Worcestershire sauce
- 2 tablespoons brown sugar

Preparation

- Take the chicken and all the other ingredients and place in a baking dish.
- Cover with foil and place within a barbeque.
- Cover it, and allow to cook for 3 hours. Every hour, add 200 ml of broth and stir.

- This should be sticky and saucy.

Nutritional info:

Calories: 155

Total fat: 5.9

Saturated fat: 2.1

Cholesterol: 72 mg

Sodium: 476 mg

Potassium: 314 mg

Total Carbohydrates: 1.2 g

Protein: 22.7 g

Barbecue Chicken Wings

Preparation Time: 2 hours

Cooking Time: 3 hours

Serves: 4

Ingredients

- 1 kilo chicken wings
- 1 tablespoon olive oil
- 2 cloves garlic, chopped
- Juice of one lemon
- 4 tablespoons ketchup
- One teaspoon thyme, freshly chopped
- Fresh coriander to garnish

Preparation

- Combine all the ingredients and marinade for 2 hours.
- Place on the barbeque on low heat, and cook for 3 hours.

- Serve with a blue cheese dip.

Nutritional info

Calories: 100

Total fat: 1.8

Saturated fat: 0

Cholesterol: 44 mg

Sodium: 918 mg

Potassium: 161 mg

Total Carbohydrates: 3.2 g

Protein: 16.9 g

Chapter 5: Soups and Stews

Mushroom Lentil Barley Stew

Preparation Time: 10 minutes

Cooking Time: 4 hours

Serves: 6

Ingredients

- 4 cups beef bone broth
- 1 cup lentils
- I cup pearl barley, uncooked
- 1 cup shiitake mushrooms, sliced
- 2 cups fresh button mushrooms, sliced
- 2 tablespoons onion powder
- 1 teaspoon garlic, crushed
- 3 bay leaves
- 1 teaspoon basil, dried
- Salt and pepper to taste

Preparation

- Take a large saucepan and put in all the ingredients, being sure to stir so that everything is well combined.
- Put over low heat and allow to cook for four hours.
- Remove bay leaves before serving.

Nutritional info

Calories: 143

Total fat: 2.3

Saturated fat: 0.6

Cholesterol: 28 mg

Sodium: 70 mg

Potassium: 328 mg

Total Carbohydrates: 18.3 g

Protein: 12.0 g

Chili con Carne

Preparation Time: 10 minutes

Cooking Time: 4 hours 30 minutes

Serves: 4

Ingredients

- ¼ cup olive oil
- 500 grams minced beef
- 1 large onion, finely chopped
- 1 can red kidney beans, drained
- 3 cups beef bone stock
- 1 can tomatoes, chopped
- 1 teaspoon cumin, ground
- Salt and pepper to taste

Preparation

- Heat up the olive oil.
- Add the beef and onion, allowing to cook until beef is well browned.

- Simmer all ingredients for 4 hours, stirring occasionally to prevent sticking.
- Serve with fragrant rice.

Nutritional info

Calories: 312

Total fat: 28.9

Saturated fat: 17.6

Cholesterol: 106 mg

Sodium: 38 mg

Potassium: 235 mg

Total Carbohydrates: 0.7 g

Protein: 12.8 g

French Onion Soup

Preparation Time: 10 minutes

Cooking Time: 8 hours 30 minutes

Serves: 4

Ingredients

- 3 tablespoons of butter
- 4 large onions, thinly sliced
- 1/4 teaspoon dried thyme
- 1 tablespoon white sugar
- 7 cups beef bone broth
- 2 cloves garlic, minced
- 1/3 cup sherry
- 1/3 cup Gruyere cheese, grated
- ¼ cup Elemental cheese, grated
- ¼ cup Mozzarella cheese, grated
- 1 tablespoon Parmesan cheese, fresh shavings
- 1 bay leaf
- 4 French bread, slices

Preparation

- Add butter and heat in the onions, sauté until transparent, around 10 minutes.
- Add sugar, reduce heat and continue cooking for 30 minutes until caramelized.
- Add garlic and cook for one minute.
- Deglaze the pan by adding sherry.
- Pour in beef bone broth and thyme, and leave to simmer on low heat for 8 hours.
- Spoon into soup bowls until ¾ full.
- Sprinkle with each of the four kinds of cheese.
- Place in a heated oven for 5 minutes, until the cheese has started to melt and bubble.
- Serve.

Nutritional info

Calories: 67

Total fat: 2.0

Saturated fat: 0.8

Cholesterol: 28 mg

Sodium: 293 mg

Potassium: 173 mg

Total Carbohydrates: 2.1 g

Protein: 9.8 g

Slow Cooker Ground Beef Stew

Preparation Time: 10 minutes

Cooking Time: 8 hours

Serves: 6

Ingredients

- Olive Oil
- 500 grams mined meat, lean
- One onion, finely chopped
- 2 cloves garlic, sliced
- One cup beef bone broth
- One cup cream of mushroom soup
- One cup tomato juice
- 1 teaspoon Worcestershire sauce
- 1 tablespoon Sherry Wine
- 5 potatoes, diced
- One cup mushrooms, sliced
- One cup peas
- One cup carrots, sliced
- One can corn, drained

- ½ teaspoon dried thyme
- ½ teaspoon dried marjoram
- Salt and Pepper

Preparation

- In a large pan, place the olive oil over medium heat. When hot, add in the ground beef and brown.
- Add all the liquid ingredients and cook.
- Add the vegetables and herbs, combine well and reduce the heat.
- Cook over a period of 8 hours until the sauce becomes thick.

Nutritional info:

Calories: 136

Total fat: 4.8

Saturated fat: 0.8

Cholesterol: 45 mg

Sodium: 340 mg

Potassium: 246 mg

Total Carbohydrates: 3.5 g

Protein: 19.3 g

Beef, Rustic Style Stew

Preparation Time: 20 minutes

Cooking Time: 6 hours 30 minutes

Serves: 8

Ingredients

- 1.5 kilos chuck steak, beef
- 2 cups bone broth
- 2 cups red wine
- One cup of water
- 1 teaspoon ground mustard seed
- 1 teaspoon dried thyme
- 4 potatoes, diced
- 3 carrots, diced
- 10 cocktail onions, diced
- Salt and Pepper

Preparation

- Take the beef and season it. Place onto a pan on high heat. Allow to brown on both sides. Set it aside.
- Take a slow cooker and put in all the other ingredients. Return the beef and cover for 6 hours, cooking on low heat.

Nutritional info

Calories: 82

Total fat: 1.6

Saturated fat: 0

Cholesterol: 37 mg

Sodium: 48 mg

Potassium: 208 mg

Total Carbohydrates: 1.9 g

Protein: 14.8 g

Minestrone Soup

Preparation Time: 20 minutes

Cooking Time: 6 hours 30 minutes

Serves: 8

Ingredients

- 1 can of diced tomatoes
- 2 cups of chopped carrots
- 2 cups of chopped potatoes
- 1.5 cups of chopped celery
- 3 cloves garlic, minced
- 1 white onion, diced
- 1 tablespoon of Italian seasoning
- 2 bay leaves
- 6 cups bone broth
- 2 cups tomato juice
- One can of cannellini beans
- One cup of cooked red kidney beans
- 3 zucchinis, diced
- One cup of tubular pasta
- One cup steamed green bean

Preparation

- Place the diced tomatoes, potatoes, carrots, celery, white onion, garlic, Italian seasoning, salt, pepper, bay leaves into a large slow cooker
- Add in the broth and the tomato juice
- Cover and leave on low heat for 6hours.
- Add in the different beans, pasta, and zucchini. Boil for 15 more minutes until pasta is cooked.

Nutritional info

Calories: 47

Total fat: 0.9

Saturated fat: 0

Cholesterol: 19 mg

Sodium: 322 mg

Potassium: 156 mg

Total Carbohydrates: 2.0 g

Protein: 7.8 g

Special Slow Beef Stew

Preparation Time: 10 minutes

Cooking Time: 7 hours

Serves: 8

Ingredients

- 1.5 kg cubed steak (beef)
- 3 carrots, chopped
- 3 stalks celery, chopped
- 2 potatoes, peeled and cubed
- 1 cup sliced fresh mushrooms
- 1 onion, chopped
- One pack onion soup
- One can mushroom soup
- 2 cups beef bone broth

Preparation

- In a slow cooker, place the vegetable

- Place the meat on top of it, and then top up with the liquids. Leave on the cooker on a low setting for 7 hours.
- If necessary, the top of the stock through the course of the day.

Nutritional info

Calories: 47

Total fat: 0.6

Saturated fat: 0

Cholesterol: 8 mg

Sodium: 52 mg

Potassium: 151 mg

Total Carbohydrates: 7.0 g

Protein: 4.0 g

Creamy Potato Soup

Preparation Time: 10 minutes

Cooking Time: 1 hour

Serves: 8

Ingredients

- 5 rashers thick cut bacon, chopped into large pieces
- 4 cups of chicken bone broth
- 1 onion, finely chopped
- 4 potatoes, diced
- 1 cup cream
- 1 cup milk
- Salt and pepper

Preparation

- Add the onion and sauté till transparent. Remove from the pan.
- In a slow-cooked, place all the other ingredients. Return the bacon to the pan.
- For 1 hour cook and serve.

94

Nutritional info

Calories: 78

Total fat: 1.5

Saturated fat: 0

Cholesterol: 33 mg

Sodium: 44 mg

Potassium: 238 mg

Total Carbohydrates: 3.0 g

Protein: 13.2 g

Chicken Taco Soup

Preparation Time: 10 minutes

Cooking Time: 3 hours

Serves: 4

Ingredients

- 4 chicken breasts, boneless and skinless
- 1 onion, finely chopped
- 1 can black beans
- 1 can corn
- 3 cans tomatoes, chopped
- 300 ml beer
- 1 teaspoon taco seasoning
- 1 Avocado, thinly sliced
- 100 gm cheddar cheese, grated
- Dash of sour cream

Preparation

- Place a large heavy bottomed saucepan over medium heat. Place the onion, beans, corn, beer, seasoning, and tomatoes in the pan. Stir well and bring to the boil.

- Add in the chicken breasts and cover, leaving to simmer on low heat for 2 hours.
- Shred the chicken, then return to the stove for one more hour.
- Serve in taco shells and sprinkle with cheddar cheese, avocado and sour cream for the garnish.

Nutritional info

Calories: 130

Total fat: 5.1

Saturated fat: 1.8

Cholesterol: 51 mg

Sodium: 437 mg

Potassium: 287 mg

Total Carbohydrates: 3.4 g

Protein: 17.5 g

Chapter 6: Side Dishes

Raw Bone Broth Cheesecake

Preparation Time: 10 minutes

Cooking Time: 3 hours

Serves: 4

Ingredients

- 2 cups almonds, cashews or nut of choice

- 1 cup pitted dates

- 4 eggs separated from whites (room temperature)

- 1 ¼ cup raw milk OR use coconut milk

- 2 tablespoons bone broth marrow OR bone broth gelatin

- ½ cup raw honey OR a tablespoon of Swerve if low carb

- 1 tablespoon vanilla

- A little salt.

Preparations

- Consider first making your nuts crispy (preferably almonds) by soaking in water for about 7 hours, drain, and place in a warm oven (150 F) for 12-18 hours.

- Process together nuts dates until homogenous.

- Press the mass into a 9 x 13 Pyrex dish, creating a crust.

- Whisk egg yolks, milk, bone marrow or gelatin, until dissolved.

- Using food processor, combine cream cheese, honey, and vanilla until smooth. Transfer to a bowl.

- Beat egg whites until stiff then fold into cream cheese mixture.

- Layer both ingredients together into crust one at a time. Chill and serve

Nutritional info

Calories: 124

Total fat: 2.6

Saturated fat: 0.8

Cholesterol: 52 mg

Sodium: 53 mg

Potassium: 267 mg

Total Carbohydrates: 4.5 g

Protein: 20.0 g

Dairy Free Raw Batter Ice Cream

Preparation Time: 10 minutes

Cooking Time: 3 hours

Serves: 4

Ingredients

- 1 15 oz can full-fat coconut milk

- 1.5 scoops bone broth protein powder

- 1/3rd cup of raw honey

- 1/3rd cup almond flour

- 1/4th teaspoon baking soda

- Optional: 2 tbsp coconut oil

Preparations

- Blend in a blender until it's a smooth mass.

- Freeze in popsicle trays.

- Or turn into cakes by baking in muffin tray for 15-20 minutes at 400 F.

Nutritional info

Calories: 114

Total fat: 3.1

Saturated fat: 1.2

Cholesterol: 43 mg

Sodium: 377 mg

Potassium: 276 mg

Total Carbohydrates: 5.3 g

Protein: 15.5 g

Baked Beans

Preparation Time: 5 minutes

Cooking Time: 2 hours

Serves: 4

Ingredients

- 3 tablespoons barbeque sauce
- 3 tablespoons packed brown sugar
- 1/2 cup ketchup
- 1 teaspoon dry mustard
- 200 grams ham, diced
- 1 large onion, finely chopped

Preparation

- Combine all the ingredients in a baking dish.
- Place on low heat in an oven pre-heated to 180 degrees C for 2 hours.

Nutritional info

Calories: 86

Total fat: 0.8

Saturated fat: 0

Cholesterol: 14 mg

Sodium: 29 mg

Potassium: 152 mg

Total Carbohydrates: 12.8 g

Protein: 7.1 g

Slow Cooker Creamed Corn

Preparation Time: 5 minutes

Cooking Time: 2 hours

Serves: 4

Ingredients

- 300 grams of frozen corn kernels, thawed
- 200 grams of cream cheese
- ½ cup milk
- 3 tablespoons butter
- 1 tablespoon sugar
- Salt and Pepper to season

Preparation

- Combine the corn, cream cheese, butter, milk, and sugar.
- Cook on low heat for two hours.
- Season with salt and pepper to taste.

Nutritional info

Calories: 258

Total fat: 8.2

Saturated fat: 2.6

Cholesterol: 112 mg

Sodium: 882 mg

Potassium: 542 mg

Total Carbohydrates: 4.7 g

Protein: 39.2 g

Casserole with Sweet Potato

Preparation Time: 15 minutes

Cooking Time: 2 hours 30 minutes

Serves: 4

Ingredients

- 600 grams sweet potato, chopped into pieces
- 4 tablespoons butter, melted
- ½ cup brown sugar
- ¼ cup orange juice
- ½ cup milk
- 2 eggs, beaten
- 2 tablespoons chopped pecans
- 3 tablespoons plain flour

Preparation

- Preheat oven to 180 degrees C
- In a large pan, place the sweet potato, lightly seasoned with salt and pepper and boil for thirty minutes.

- Add the melted butter and sugar and cook until heated through. Mash in the pan.
- Add in the orange juice, milk, and eggs. Transfer this mixture into a lightly greased baking dish.
- In a small bowl, mix the pecans, brown sugar, butter, and flour. Place this mixture over the sweet potatoes.
- Bake for two hours, until the top, is crusty.

Nutritional info

Calories: 106

Total fat: 2.0

Saturated fat: 0.6

Cholesterol: 43 mg

Sodium: 46 mg

Potassium: 288 mg

Total Carbohydrates: 5.3 g

Protein: 16.3 g

Baked Potatoes

Preparation Time: 5 minutes

Cooking Time: 2 hours

Serves: 4

Ingredients

- 4 sheets of aluminum foil
- 4 baking potatoes unpeeled and scrubbed
- 1 tablespoon olive oil
- Salt and pepper to season

Preparation

- Poke the potatoes with a fork and rub with the olive oil.
- Season and wrap with foil.
- Bake for 2 hours.
- Serve with a variety of accompaniments, such as cream cheese.

Nutritional info

Calories: 124

Total fat: 2.6

Saturated fat: 0.8

Cholesterol: 52 mg

Sodium: 53 mg

Potassium: 267 mg

Total Carbohydrates: 4.5 g

Protein: 20.0 g

Slow Cooker Beans

Preparation Time: Overnight

Cooking Time: 4 hours

Serves: 4

Ingredients

- 7 cups beef bone broth
- 1 tablespoon olive oil
- 1 kg dry beans
- 1 small onion, finely chopped
- 2 teaspoons onion and garlic powder
- 3 bay leaves
- 100 grams smoked turkey

Preparation

- Pick the beans, and clean them. Soak them overnight in cool water.
- Cover with the stock and other ingredients and stir after draining.
- Cook on a slow cooked for 4 hours.

- Serve, when beans are tender.

Garlic Mashed Potatoes

Preparation Time: Overnight

Cooking Time: 1 hour

Serves: 4

Ingredients

- 1-kilo potatoes, diced
- 2 cups chicken bone broth
- 100 grams cream cheese
- 1 teaspoon garlic, crushed
- Salt and Pepper
- A dollop of butter

Preparation

- Preheat the oven to 180 degrees C
- Put the potatoes into a saucepan and cover with chicken broth and boil.
- When tender, after 20 minutes, drain and place in a bowl.

- Mash until creamy.
- Place mashed potatoes into the oven for 40 minutes until there is a light brown crust.

Nutritional info

Calories: 80

Total fat: 1.6

Saturated fat: 0.6

Cholesterol: 22 mg

Sodium: 317 mg

Potassium: 172 mg

Total Carbohydrates: 3.0 g

Protein: 7.9 g

Mashed Potatoes

Preparation Time: 5 minutes

Cooking Time: 1 hours

Serves: 4

Ingredients

- 2 potatoes, cut into chunks
- 2 cloves garlic, minced
- ¼ cup chicken bone broth
- 1 tablespoon sour cream
- Butter, salt and pepper to taste

Preparation

- Boil the potatoes until soft. Drain and place in a large bowl.
- Mash potatoes with all the other ingredients until smooth.
- Transfer the potato mixture into a baking dish and place in oven for 1 hour.

Bone Broth Custard

Preparation Time: 10 minutes

Cooking Time: 35 minutes

Serves: 6

Ingredients

- 3 pounds beef marrow bones

- ¾ cup milk or coconut milk

- 1 tablespoon vanilla extract

- 2 tablespoon honey

- ¼ tablespoon Himalayan salt

- Coconut oil for greasing

Preparation

- Let marrow/bones boil and simmer for 10 minutes. Preheat oven to 350 f

- Mix all ingredients together in a bowl.

- When marrow is ready, scoop with a slotted spoon. Place in bowl to drain.

- Mix with the rest of the ingredients and add to an immersion blender. Blend.

- Now, pour into custard baking cups and bake for 35 minutes, until custards are set in the center.

Nutritional info

Calories: 124

Total fat: 2.6

Saturated fat: 0.8

Cholesterol: 52 mg

Sodium: 53 mg

Potassium: 267 mg

Total Carbohydrates: 4.5 g

Protein: 20.0 g

Creamed Spinach

Preparation Time: 5 minutes

Cooking Time: 1 hour

Serves: 4

Ingredient

- 100 grams fresh spinach, chopped
- 2 cups cottage cheese
- 2 tablespoons butter
- 1 egg, beaten
- Salt and pepper to taste

Preparation

- Get a medium sized, heavy based pan. Combine all the ingredients in the pan, making sure that they mix well.
- Place on low heat and allow to cook gently for one hour. Make sure you stir to prevent sticking.

Collard Greens

Preparation Time: 10 minutes

Cooking Time: 2 hours

Serves: 4

Ingredients

- 4 bunches of collard greens. Rinsed, trimmed and chopped
- 1 cup of chicken bone broth
- 150 grams ham shanks
- 4 pickled jalapeno peppers, roughly chopped
- 1 garlic clove, sliced
- 1/2 teaspoon baking soda
- 1 teaspoon olive oil
- Ground black pepper to taste

Preparation

- Place the ham shanks into the broth, and top up with collard greens. Bring to a gentle boil.
- Once the greens start wilting, add in the rest of the ingredients.
- Alternate layers of greens with the ham shanks and jalapeno until the slow cooker is full.
- Cover, and then reduce heat to Low. Cook for 2 hours.

Nutritional info:

Calories: 114

Total fat: 3.1

Saturated fat: 1.2

Cholesterol: 43 mg

Sodium: 377 mg

Potassium: 276 mg

Total Carbohydrates: 5.3 g

Protein: 15.5 g

Spiced Applesauce

Preparation Time: 5 minutes

Cooking Time: 1 hour

Serves: 4

Ingredients

- 8 apples peeled, cored, and chopped
- One cup of water
- Pinch of cinnamon
- ½ cup brown sugar

Preparation

- Take a medium saucepan and place all the ingredients within it.
- Cover and simmer on low heat for 1 hour. Blend and serve.

Nutritional info

Calories: 69

Total fat: 2.0

Saturated fat: 0.6

Cholesterol: 21 mg

Sodium: 431 mg

Potassium: 286 mg

Total Carbohydrates: 5.7 g

Protein: 7.8 g

Conclusion

As you have seen in the recipe chapter, each recipe has been presented with the number of servings. The advantage of having a meal plan is that you know ahead what your week is going to look like. As you decide on the things that you are going to eat and you prepare the bone broth in advance, you have a reduce chance of falling prey to temptations.

Once you have added the desired recipes to your meal plan, the next step will be to print it out and display it in the kitchen. This will help you stick to the bone broth diet, allowing you to follow the established pattern and finally achieve the desired weight. And, remember, the bone broth diet is not only about losing weight but also about making healthier eating choices. No faster or junk foods, no more sugary drinks and no more refined fats. You will come to love bone broth, as it is highly nutritious and easy-to-prepare.

www.ingramcontent.com/pod-product-compliance
Lightning Source LLC
Chambersburg PA
CBHW072055280526
45788CB00006B/2295